From Bites to Battles: The Ongoing Fight Against Lyme Disease.

All rights reserved. No part of this publication may be reproduced, distributed, or transmitted in any form or by any means, including photocopying, recording, or other electronic or mechanical methods, without the prior written permission of the publisher, except in the case of brief quotations embodied in critical reviews and certain other noncommercial uses permitted by copyright law.

Copyright © (Dr.Barry Young), (2024).

Table of Contents.

INTRODUCTION.

Chapter 1.
Causes and Transmission.

Chapter 2.
Symptoms and Stages.

Chapter 3.
Diagnosis.

Chapter 4.
Prevention.

Chapter 5.

Research and Developments.

Chapter 6.

Impact on Society.

Chapter 7.

Controversies and Debates.

INTRODUCTION.

Lyme disease, a multisystem infectious disease, is caused by the spirochete bacterium "Borrelia burgdorferi". Transmitted primarily through the bites of infected black-legged ticks, Lyme disease affects numerous bodily systems, leading to a wide array of symptoms.

This introduction explores the historical context of Lyme disease and identifies the regions where it is most prevalent.

The history of Lyme disease dates back to the early 20th century, although the condition was not formally recognized until much later.

Early Observations:

As early as the 1900s, European physicians reported cases of a skin rash later recognized as erythema migrans, a hallmark of early Lyme disease. These observations laid the groundwork for understanding the dermatological aspects of the disease.

The disease is named after the town of Old Lyme, Connecticut, where in the mid-1970s, a cluster of children and adults experienced unusual arthritic symptoms.

This outbreak led to the initial identification of the disease in the United States.

A pivotal moment occurred in 1975 when two mothers, Polly Murray and Judith Mensch, alerted health authorities about numerous cases of juvenile rheumatoid arthritis in their community.

Their observations prompted an investigation by Dr. Allen Steere and colleagues, who identified the condition as a distinct entity, later named Lyme arthritis.

Identification of the Causative Agent:

In 1981, Dr. Willy Burgdorfer, a medical entomologist, discovered the bacterium "Borrelia burgdorferi" in the midgut of Ixodes ticks.

This groundbreaking discovery confirmed the bacterial etiology of Lyme disease and identified ticks as vectors.

Dr. Burgdorfer's discovery was a significant milestone in medical science, earning widespread recognition and highlighting the importance of vector-borne diseases.

Further Research and Developments:

- Evolution of Diagnostics and Treatment: Following the identification of Borrelia burgdorferi extensive research focused on improving diagnostic methods and developing effective treatments. Advances in molecular biology and immunology have enhanced our understanding of the disease's pathogenesis and immune response.

- Continued Surveillance: Ongoing surveillance and research continue to refine our knowledge of Lyme disease, including its epidemiology, clinical manifestations, and long-term outcomes.

Regions Most Affected by Lyme Disease.

Lyme disease is a global concern, but its prevalence varies significantly across different regions. Understanding the geographic distribution of Lyme disease is crucial for public health efforts and preventive measures.

North America:

-United States: Lyme disease is most prevalent in the northeastern, mid-Atlantic, and north-central regions of the United States. States such as Connecticut, Massachusetts, New York, New Jersey, Pennsylvania, Wisconsin, and

Minnesota report the highest incidence rates. The Centers for Disease Control and Prevention (CDC) estimates that approximately 476,000 Americans are diagnosed and treated for Lyme disease annually.

Canada: In Canada, Lyme disease cases have increased in recent years, particularly in southern regions of British Columbia, Manitoba, Ontario, Quebec, and the Atlantic provinces.

The expansion of tick habitats due to climate change and other ecological factors contributes to this rise.

Europe:

- Western Europe: Lyme disease is endemic in several European countries, including Germany, Austria, Slovenia, and the Scandinavian nations. The incidence rates vary, with some areas reporting significant numbers of cases. The European Centre for Disease Prevention and Control (ECDC) monitors Lyme disease across the continent, highlighting the need for awareness and preventive measures.

- Central and Eastern Europe.

Countries such as Poland, Czech Republic, and Slovakia also experience high rates of Lyme disease. The diverse landscapes and tick habitats in these regions contribute to the widespread nature of the disease.

Asia:

Northeast Asia: In Asia, Lyme disease is reported in northeastern regions, including parts of Russia, China, and Japan. The disease's prevalence in these areas underscores the importance of international collaboration in research and surveillance.

Environmental and Climatic Factors.

- Tick Habitats: The distribution of Lyme disease correlates with the habitats of tick vectors, primarily the Ixodes species. Forested and grassy areas with abundant wildlife hosts, such as deer and rodents, provide ideal environments for ticks.

- Climate Change: Climate change significantly impacts the spread of Lyme disease by altering tick habitats and extending their active seasons. Warmer temperatures and changing precipitation patterns contribute to the northward expansion of tick populations, increasing the risk of Lyme disease in previously unaffected areas.

Lyme disease's history, from its early recognition to the discovery of its causative agent, underscores the importance of scientific inquiry and public health vigilance.

Understanding the regions most affected by Lyme disease highlights the need for targeted prevention and awareness efforts.

As research continues to evolve, it is crucial to remain vigilant and proactive in combating this persistent and potentially debilitating diseases.

Chapter 1.

Causes and Transmission.

Lyme disease is caused by the bacterium "Borrelia burgdorferi" and is primarily transmitted to humans through the bites of infected ticks.

The Role of Borrelia burgdorferi.

Borrelia burgdorferi is a spiral-shaped bacterium belonging to the spirochete family. It is the causative agent of Lyme disease and is primarily found in the midgut of certain species of ticks, particularly those belonging to the genus *Ixodes*.

The life cycle of Borrelia burgdorferi involves complex interactions between ticks, reservoir hosts (such as rodents and small mammals), and humans.

Here's a detailed look at the role of "Borrelia burgdorferi" in the transmission of Lyme disease:

Borrelia burgdorferi is acquired by ticks during their blood meal from infected reservoir hosts. Small mammals, such as white-footed mice and chipmunks, serve as the primary reservoirs for the bacterium in endemic areas.

Once ingested, Borrelia burgdorferi colonizes the midgut of the tick and undergoes a series of developmental stages, including replication and migration to the salivary glands.

When an infected tick bites a human host, the bacterium is transmitted through the tick's saliva into the bloodstream. The transmission process is facilitated by the tick's feeding behavior, which involves prolonged attachment to the host.

How Ticks Spread Lyme Disease.

Ticks play a critical role in the spread of Lyme disease, acting as vectors for the transmission of *Borrelia burgdorferi* to humans.

Understanding the mechanisms by which ticks spread Lyme disease is essential for developing effective prevention strategies. Here's an overview of how ticks transmit Lyme disease:

Ticks have a specialized feeding behavior that enables them to obtain a blood meal from their hosts. During feeding, ticks secrete saliva containing a complex mixture of bioactive compounds, including anticoagulants and immunomodulatory factors.

As ticks feed, they inject saliva into the host's bloodstream to facilitate blood uptake. If the tick is infected with Borrelia burgdorferi, the bacterium is also introduced into the host's bloodstream along with the saliva.

Once in the host's bloodstream, Borrelia burgdorferi interacts with the host's immune system. The bacterium has evolved various mechanisms to evade immune detection and establish infection in the host's tissues.

Borrelia burgdorferi disseminates from the site of the tick bite to various tissues and organs, leading to the characteristic clinical manifestations of Lyme disease. The bacterium can infect the skin, joints, heart, and nervous system, causing a wide range of symptoms.

Identifying Tick Species Responsible for Lyme Disease.

Not all tick species are capable of transmitting Lyme disease, and the identification of tick species responsible for its transmission is crucial for understanding disease epidemiology and implementing targeted control measures. The primary tick vectors implicated in the transmission of Lyme disease belong to the genus "Ixodes", with specific species playing prominent roles in different regions. Here's a closer look at the tick species responsible for Lyme disease transmission:

Ixodes scapularis (Black-legged Tick) Commonly known as the black-legged tick or deer tick, "Ixodes scapularis" is the primary vector of Lyme disease in the northeastern and north-central United States.

This tick species feeds on a variety of hosts, including mammals, birds, and reptiles, and is responsible for the majority of Lyme disease cases in the United States.

Ixodes pacificus (Western Black-legged Tick) Ixodes pacificus is the primary vector of Lyme disease on the Pacific coast of the United States, particularly in California and Oregon.

This tick species feeds on similar hosts as Ixodes scapularis and contributes to the geographic distribution of Lyme disease in western regions.

Ixodes ricinus (European Sheep Tick) In Europe, Ixodes ricinus is the principal vector of Lyme disease, transmitting Borrelia burgdorferi to humans and animals across various European countries.

This tick species is commonly found in wooded and grassy areas and feeds on a wide range of hosts, including rodents, deer, and birds.

Understanding the causes and transmission of Lyme disease is fundamental to its prevention and control. "Borrelia burgdorferi" plays a central role as the causative agent, while ticks serve as vectors for its transmission to humans.

By identifying the tick species responsible for Lyme disease transmission and studying their biology and ecology, public health authorities can implement targeted interventions to reduce the burden of this debilitating disease.

Chapter 2.

Symptoms and Stages.

Lyme disease is known for its varied symptoms, which can affect multiple systems in the body and present in distinct stages. Understanding these symptoms and stages is crucial for timely diagnosis and treatment. This section will cover the early indicators, progression of the disease, and the ongoing debate surrounding chronic Lyme disease.

The early stage of Lyme disease, often called localized Lyme disease, typically manifests within 3 to 30 days after a tick bite.

Recognizing these initial symptoms is critical for early diagnosis and effective treatment.

- Erythema Migrans (EM) Rash: The EM rash is one of the hallmark symptoms of early Lyme disease. It typically appears at the site of the tick bite and gradually expands over several days. The rash often has a characteristic "bull's-eye" appearance with a red outer ring surrounding a central clear area, but it can also appear uniformly red. The EM rash is usually not painful or itchy, which can sometimes delay its recognition.

- Flu-like Symptoms: Many patients experience flu-like symptoms, including fever, chills, headache, fatigue, muscle and joint aches, and swollen lymph nodes. These symptoms can be nonspecific and similar to other viral infections, which may complicate early diagnosis.

- Other Early Symptoms: Some patients may experience additional symptoms such as neck stiffness, sensitivity to light (photophobia), and conjunctivitis (eye inflammation).

Recognizing these early indicators and seeking medical attention promptly is crucial, as early treatment with antibiotics can prevent the progression of Lyme disease.

Progression of the Disease: Advanced Symptoms.

If Lyme disease is not diagnosed and treated in its early stages, the infection can spread to other parts of the body, leading to more severe and diverse symptoms. This stage is often referred to as disseminated Lyme disease and can occur weeks to months after the initial tick bite.

As the bacteria disseminate, multiple EM rashes may appear on different parts of the body. These secondary rashes may not have the classic bull's-eye appearance.

Neurological Symptoms (Neuroborreliosis):

Neurological involvement can occur in approximately 10-15% of untreated patients.

Symptoms include facial palsy (loss of muscle tone or droop on one or both sides of the face), meningitis (severe headaches, neck stiffness, sensitivity to light), and radiculoneuritis (sharp shooting pains, numbness, or tingling in the limbs).

Cardiac Symptoms (Lyme Carditis):

Lyme carditis can cause palpitations, chest pain, and shortness of breath.Some patients may develop heart block, a serious condition where the electrical signals in the heart are disrupted, requiring immediate medical attention.

Musculoskeletal Symptoms:

Joint pain and swelling, particularly in the large joints such as the knees, are common in disseminated Lyme disease. These symptoms can be intermittent and may affect different joints at different times.

Other Systemic Symptoms:

Fatigue, which can be profound and persistent. Additional symptoms may include dizziness, shortness of breath, and mood changes such as irritability or depression.

The progression of Lyme disease can be insidious, and the variability in symptoms underscores the importance of considering Lyme disease in differential diagnosis when patients present with compatible symptoms, especially in endemic areas.

The concept of chronic Lyme disease is highly controversial and has sparked considerable debate among medical professionals, researchers, and patient advocacy groups. Here, we explore the arguments and evidence on both sides of the debate.

Chronic Lyme disease, sometimes referred to as Post-Treatment Lyme Disease Syndrome (PTLDS), describes a condition where patients continue to experience symptoms such as fatigue, pain, and cognitive difficulties for months or years after completing antibiotic treatment.

Symptoms are often subjective and can significantly impact quality of life.

Arguments Supporting Chronic Lyme Disease:

- Proponents argue that *Borrelia burgdorferi* can persist in the body despite antibiotic treatment, potentially leading to ongoing symptoms.

- Some studies have identified evidence of persistent infection in animal models and, to a lesser extent, in humans.

- Patients and advocacy groups emphasize the real and debilitating nature of their symptoms, calling for further research and validation of chronic Lyme disease.

Arguments Against Chronic Lyme Disease:

- Many medical professionals and organizations, including the Infectious Diseases Society of America (IDSA), question the existence of chronic Lyme disease, attributing persistent symptoms to other causes such as autoimmune reactions, co-infections, or other undiagnosed conditions.

- Controlled studies have shown that prolonged antibiotic therapy does not significantly improve long-term outcomes for patients with persistent symptoms after standard treatment.

- Critics argue that the term "chronic Lyme disease" may lead to unnecessary and potentially harmful treatments.

Current Consensus and Ongoing Research:

There is consensus that a subset of patients experience persistent symptoms after Lyme disease treatment, but the exact cause and appropriate management remain areas of active research.

Research continues to explore the mechanisms behind PTLDS, including potential immune system involvement, persistence of bacterial remnants, and other biological factors.

Understanding the symptoms and stages of Lyme disease is vital for effective diagnosis and treatment. Early recognition of initial symptoms can lead to prompt treatment and better outcomes, while awareness of the progression to advanced symptoms highlights the need for timely medical intervention.

The debate over chronic Lyme disease underscores the complexities and challenges in managing this multifaceted condition, emphasizing the need for continued research and patient-centered care.

Chapter 3.

Diagnosis.

Diagnosing Lyme disease can be challenging due to its varied symptoms and the limitations of current testing methods. This section covers the key aspects of diagnosing Lyme disease, including clinical evaluation and blood tests, the challenges in achieving an accurate diagnosis, and the importance of early detection.

Diagnosing Lyme disease typically involves a combination of clinical evaluation and laboratory testing.

Here's a detailed overview of the process:

- Clinical Evaluation:

A thorough medical history and physical examination are crucial. Physicians look for characteristic symptoms such as erythema migrans (EM) rash, flu-like symptoms, and potential exposure to tick habitats. Evaluating the likelihood of tick exposure based on the patient's activities and geographic location helps assess risk.

Clinicians examine the skin for the EM rash and assess for signs of neurological, cardiac, and musculoskeletal involvement.

- Blood Tests:

Two-Tiered Testing Approach: The standard laboratory diagnosis for Lyme disease involves a two-tiered testing approach.

ELISA (Enzyme-Linked Immunosorbent Assay): This initial test detects antibodies against Borrelia burgdorferi. A positive or equivocal result leads to a confirmatory test.

This confirmatory test further examines the presence of specific antibodies against Borrelia burgdorferi. The IgM and IgG antibody responses are evaluated separately.

Antibodies typically take several weeks to develop, so testing too early after exposure may result in false negatives. Testing is most reliable a few weeks after the onset of symptoms.

Accurate diagnosis of Lyme disease presents several challenges due to the complex nature of the disease and limitations of current diagnostic tools:

Early symptoms of Lyme disease, such as fever, fatigue, and muscle aches, overlap with many other illnesses, making clinical diagnosis difficult without the presence of the EM rash.

The absence of a visible tick bite or rash can further complicate diagnosis, as many patients do not recall being bitten.

Limitations of Serological Tests:

Early in the infection, patients may not yet have developed detectable levels of antibodies, leading to false-negative results.Cross-reactivity with antibodies from other infections can result in false-positive results, particularly in areas where other tick-borne illnesses are prevalent.

Even after successful treatment, antibodies can persist in the bloodstream for months or years, complicating the interpretation of test results.

The accuracy of tests can vary depending on the stage of the disease and the quality of the testing procedures. Laboratory standards and experience also play a role in test reliability.

Patients with chronic symptoms may suffer from co-infections with other tick-borne pathogens, which can complicate the diagnostic picture and require additional testing.

Importance of Early Detection.

Early detection and treatment of Lyme disease are crucial for preventing severe complications and long-term health issues:

Early detection allows for prompt treatment with antibiotics, which can effectively eliminate *Borrelia burgdorferi* and prevent the bacteria from spreading to other parts of the body.

Timely intervention can prevent the development of more severe symptoms such as Lyme arthritis, neurological disorders, and Lyme carditis.

Early treatment significantly reduces the risk of persistent symptoms that can occur if the disease progresses untreated. This includes reducing the likelihood of developing Post-Treatment Lyme Disease Syndrome (PTLDS).

Prompt diagnosis and treatment help patients recover more quickly and avoid the physical and emotional toll of prolonged illness.

Early detection also reduces the healthcare burden by preventing complications that require more extensive and costly treatments.

Accurate diagnosis of Lyme disease relies on a combination of clinical evaluation and laboratory testing. Despite challenges such as non-specific symptoms and limitations of serological tests, early detection remains critical for effective treatment and prevention of severe complications.

Continued advancements in diagnostic methods and greater awareness among healthcare providers and the public are essential to improving outcomes for patients with Lyme disease.

Chapter 4.

Prevention.

Preventing Lyme disease involves a combination of personal protection measures, effective tick removal techniques, and public health initiatives to raise awareness and educate communities. This section explores strategies to protect against tick bites, methods for safely removing ticks, and the role of public health campaigns in Lyme disease prevention.

The primary way to prevent Lyme disease is to avoid tick bites, especially in areas known for high tick activity.

Here are detailed strategies to protect yourself:

When hiking or walking in wooded or grassy areas, stick to the center of trails to avoid brushing against vegetation where ticks may be waiting.

Ticks are commonly found in tall grass, brush, and leaf litter. Avoid these areas when possible.

Wear long-sleeved shirts and long pants to minimize exposed skin. Tuck pants into socks or boots to prevent ticks from crawling up your legs. Wear light-colored clothing to make it easier to spot ticks.

Use EPA-registered insect repellents containing DEET, picaridin, IR3535, or oil of lemon eucalyptus on exposed skin. Follow product instructions for safe use.

Treat clothing and gear, such as boots, pants, and socks, with permethrin, an insecticide that kills ticks on contact. Pre-treated clothing is also available for purchase.

Check your body for ticks after spending time outdoors. Pay special attention to areas where ticks are commonly found, such as the armpits, groin, back of the knees, scalp, and waistband.

Take a shower soon after being outdoors to wash off unattached ticks and make it easier to spot any ticks that may be attached.

Use veterinarian-recommended tick prevention products on pets. Pets can bring ticks into the home, increasing the risk of tick bites for humans. Inspect pets for ticks regularly, especially after they have been outdoors.

Effective Tick Removal Techniques.

Even with preventive measures, tick bites can still occur. Proper and prompt removal of attached ticks is crucial to reduce the risk of Lyme disease transmission.

- Use fine-tipped tweezers to grasp the tick as close to the skin's surface as possible.

- Pull upward with steady, even pressure. Avoid twisting or jerking, which can cause the mouthparts to break off and remain in the skin.

- Clean the bite area and your hands with rubbing alcohol, an iodine scrub, or soap and water.

- Dispose of the tick by placing it in alcohol, sealing it in a bag, wrapping it tightly in tape, or flushing it down the toilet. Do not crush the tick with your fingers.

+ After removing a tick, monitor for any symptoms of Lyme disease, such as rash, fever, chills, fatigue, muscle aches, or joint pain.

+ If you develop symptoms or are concerned about the risk of Lyme disease, contact a healthcare provider.

Public Health Campaigns and Awareness.

Public health campaigns play a vital role in preventing Lyme disease by raising awareness and educating communities about the risks and prevention strategies.

Public health agencies conduct outreach programs to educate communities about tick-borne diseases, how to prevent tick bites, and the importance of early detection.

Schools play a critical role in educating children about tick prevention. Programs include information on avoiding tick habitats, performing tick checks, and recognizing symptoms of Lyme disease.

- Media Campaigns:

- Public Service Announcements: Television, radio, and social media campaigns disseminate information about Lyme disease prevention to a broad audience.

- Print Materials: Brochures, posters, and fact sheets distributed in healthcare facilities, parks, and community centers provide essential information on tick prevention and Lyme disease awareness.

- Collaborations with Healthcare Providers:

  • Training for Healthcare Professionals: Public health organizations provide training and resources for healthcare providers to improve the diagnosis and management of Lyme disease.

  • Reporting and Surveillance: Enhanced reporting and surveillance systems help track Lyme disease cases, identify high-risk areas, and inform targeted prevention efforts.

  • Funding Research: Public health agencies fund research to improve diagnostic methods, develop vaccines, and explore new prevention strategies.

- Policy Advocacy: Advocating for policies that support Lyme disease prevention, such as funding for public health programs and promoting land management practices that reduce tick habitats.

Preventing Lyme disease requires a multifaceted approach that includes personal protection measures, effective tick removal techniques, and robust public health campaigns.

By taking proactive steps to protect against tick bites, educating the public, and supporting research and policy initiatives, we can reduce the incidence of Lyme disease and safeguard public health.

Chapter 5.

Research and Developments.

The field of Lyme disease research is dynamic, with ongoing efforts to improve our understanding of the disease, enhance diagnostic methods, and develop effective vaccines. This section covers recent breakthroughs in Lyme disease research, innovations in diagnostic techniques, and the pursuit of a vaccine.

Recent years have seen significant advances in Lyme disease research, contributing to a better understanding of the disease's pathology, epidemiology, and potential treatments.

Advances in genomic sequencing have provided deeper insights into the genetic makeup of *Borrelia burgdorferi*. Understanding the bacterium's genome helps identify potential targets for new treatments and vaccines.

Genomic studies also reveal variations among different strains of *Borrelia*, which can influence disease presentation and severity.

Research into how *Borrelia burgdorferi* evades the immune system and persists in the human body is crucial. Studies have shown that the bacterium can alter its surface proteins to avoid detection, contributing to chronic symptoms in some patients.

Investigating the biofilm formation by *Borrelia* offers new perspectives on why some infections are resistant to treatment.

Understanding the immune response to *Borrelia burgdorferi* has led to discoveries about how the bacterium disrupts immune signaling and causes inflammation.

Research into the role of specific immune cells and cytokines in Lyme disease pathogenesis helps identify potential therapeutic targets.

Accurate and early diagnosis of Lyme disease remains a challenge, prompting ongoing research into developing more reliable and efficient diagnostic tools.

Next-generation sequencing (NGS) technologies are being explored to identify *Borrelia* DNA directly from patient samples. NGS can detect the presence of the bacterium even in low quantities, improving diagnostic accuracy.

Metagenomic sequencing allows for the simultaneous detection of multiple pathogens, which is particularly useful in diagnosing co-infections.

Novel serological tests are being developed to improve the sensitivity and specificity of antibody detection. These include tests that target different antigens or use advanced platforms such as enzyme-linked immunospot (ELISPOT) assays.

Multiplex assays, which can detect antibodies against multiple *Borrelia* proteins, offer a more comprehensive approach to diagnosis.

Point-of-care diagnostic tools, which provide rapid results at the site of patient care, are in development. These tests aim to improve accessibility and reduce the time to diagnosis, particularly in resource-limited settings.

Lateral flow assays, similar to home pregnancy tests, are being investigated for their potential to provide quick and easy Lyme disease testing.

Developing a vaccine for Lyme disease has been a high priority for researchers, given the significant public health impact of the disease.

The first Lyme disease vaccine, LYMErix, was introduced in the late 1990s but was withdrawn from the market in 2002 due to low demand and concerns about potential side effects. Despite the setback, the lessons learned from LYMErix have informed current vaccine development efforts.

- Current Vaccine Candidates:

Several new vaccine candidates are in various stages of development, targeting different components of *Borrelia burgdorferi*. These include:

*Subunit Vaccines: These vaccines use specific proteins from *Borrelia* to elicit an immune response. For example, VLA15, surface protein A (OspA) of the bacterium.

*mRNA Vaccines: Building on the success of mRNA vaccines for COVID-19, researchers are exploring mRNA platforms for Lyme disease. These vaccines can be rapidly developed and customized to target specific bacterial proteins.

*Whole-Cell Vaccines: These vaccines use inactivated or attenuated *Borrelia* cells to stimulate immunity. They aim to provide broad protection by targeting multiple antigens simultaneously.

Developing a Lyme disease vaccine faces several challenges, including the need to protect against multiple *Borrelia* species and strains, ensuring long-term immunity, and addressing potential safety concerns.

Ongoing clinical trials and research are focused on overcoming these challenges, with the goal of providing a safe and effective vaccine to the public.

The landscape of Lyme disease research and development is rapidly evolving, driven by advances in genomics, immunology, and biotechnology.

Breakthroughs in understanding the disease, innovations in diagnostic methods, and promising developments in vaccine research offer hope for better prevention, diagnosis, and treatment of Lyme disease in the future.

Continued investment in research and collaboration among scientists, healthcare providers, and public health agencies are essential to address this complex and pervasive disease effectively.

Chapter 6.

Impact on Society.

Lyme disease affects society in multifaceted ways, from economic burdens and social challenges to personal stories that highlight the human side of the illness. This section delves into the economic and social consequences, presents personal stories and case studies, and discusses public health policies and management strategies for Lyme disease.

The economic and social impacts of Lyme disease are significant and far-reaching, affecting individuals, families, and broader communities.

The direct medical costs associated with Lyme disease include expenses for doctor visits, diagnostic tests, medications, and hospitalizations. Chronic cases or complications can lead to substantial long-term medical expenses.

Indirect costs such as lost wages, reduced productivity, and disability benefits add to the economic burden. Patients with chronic symptoms may face extended periods of inability to work, impacting their financial stability.

Chronic Lyme disease can severely affect quality of life, causing persistent pain, fatigue, cognitive impairment, and emotional distress. These symptoms can hinder daily activities and social interactions, leading to isolation and depression.

The stigma and misunderstanding surrounding Lyme disease, particularly chronic Lyme disease, can exacerbate the social challenges faced by patients. Misdiagnosis or delayed diagnosis often leads to frustration and a sense of helplessness.

High incidence rates in endemic areas can strain local healthcare systems, requiring increased resources for diagnosis, treatment, and prevention efforts.

The spread of Lyme disease also impacts sectors such as tourism and outdoor recreation, as concerns about tick bites may deter people from engaging in outdoor activities.

Personal Stories and Case Studies.

Personal stories and case studies provide a human perspective on the struggles and triumphs of those affected by Lyme disease.

Case Study 1:

Jane, a 45-year-old teacher, was diagnosed with Lyme disease after experiencing persistent flu-like symptoms and joint pain. Despite initial treatment, her symptoms worsened, leading to a diagnosis of chronic Lyme disease.

Jane's journey highlights the challenges of navigating the healthcare system, dealing with skepticism from medical professionals, and managing the financial and emotional toll of long-term illness. Her story underscores the importance of patient advocacy and support networks.

Case Study 2:

Tom, a 30-year-old outdoor enthusiast, contracted Lyme disease after a camping trip. Early recognition of the classic bullseye rash led to prompt treatment with antibiotics, resulting in a full recovery.

Tom's story emphasizes the importance of early detection and awareness of Lyme disease symptoms. His experience showcases how education and quick medical intervention can lead to positive outcomes.

Case Study 3:

In a small town in Connecticut, a cluster of Lyme disease cases prompted a community-wide response. Local healthcare providers, public health officials, and residents collaborated on educational campaigns, tick control measures, and support groups for affected individuals.

This case study illustrates the power of community action in managing and mitigating the impact of Lyme disease, demonstrating how collective efforts can enhance public health and resilience.

Public Health Policy and Lyme Disease Management.

Effective management of Lyme disease requires comprehensive public health policies and strategies that encompass prevention, education, and treatment.

Robust surveillance systems are essential for tracking Lyme disease incidence and identifying emerging hotspots. Accurate reporting helps allocate resources and inform public health interventions.

Collaborations between local, state, and national health agencies improve data collection and analysis, facilitating timely and targeted responses to outbreaks.

Public health campaigns focus on educating the public about tick bite prevention, early symptom recognition, and the importance of prompt medical attention. These programs often target high-risk populations, such as outdoor workers, hikers, and children.

Schools, parks, and community organizations play a crucial role in disseminating information and promoting preventive measures.

Policies that support funding for Lyme disease research, improved diagnostic tools, and access to affordable treatment are critical. Advocacy groups often work to influence legislation and secure resources for Lyme disease initiatives.

Land management practices that reduce tick habitats, such as controlled burns and landscaping modifications, are implemented in endemic areas to lower tick populations and reduce human exposure.

ITM strategies combine biological, chemical, and environmental methods to control tick populations. This approach includes the use of acaricides, biological control agents like entomopathogenic fungi, and habitat modification.

Public health policies promoting ITM aim to reduce tick densities and interrupt the transmission cycle of Lyme disease.

The impact of Lyme disease on society is profound, encompassing economic burdens, social challenges, and public health implications. Personal stories and case studies humanize the statistics, highlighting the need for empathy, support, and comprehensive care for those affected.

Effective public health policies and management strategies are essential to address the complexities of Lyme disease, promoting prevention, early detection, and equitable access to treatment. Through continued research, education, and community collaboration, we can mitigate the impact of Lyme disease and enhance the well-being of affected individuals and communities.

Chapter 7.

Controversies and Debates.

Lyme disease is surrounded by several controversies and debates that impact patient care, treatment approaches, and public perception.

These issues are particularly pronounced in discussions about chronic Lyme disease, differing treatment methodologies, and the ethical and legal aspects of Lyme disease management. This section explores these contentious topics in detail.

The Chronic Lyme Disease Controversy.

The existence and diagnosis of chronic Lyme disease, also known as post-treatment Lyme disease syndrome (PTLDS), are highly debated within the medical community.

Proponents argue that chronic Lyme disease results from ongoing infection by *Borrelia burgdorferi*, immune system dysregulation, or persistent bacterial remnants causing inflammation.

Critics contend that there is insufficient evidence to support the idea of persistent infection and suggest that symptoms may result from an autoimmune response or other unrelated conditions.

Patients suffering from chronic symptoms often face significant challenges, including misdiagnosis, lack of recognition from healthcare providers, and limited treatment options. The controversy contributes to a sense of isolation and frustration among these patients.

Disputes Over Treatment Approaches.

Treatment of Lyme disease, particularly chronic Lyme disease, is another area of significant debate.

The standard treatment for early Lyme disease involves a course of oral antibiotics, typically doxycycline, amoxicillin, or cefuroxime, which is generally effective in most cases.

For chronic Lyme disease, some physicians advocate for prolonged antibiotic therapy, often intravenous, based on the belief that longer treatment is necessary to eradicate the infection.

However, this approach is controversial and not widely endorsed by major medical organizations due to concerns about antibiotic resistance, side effects, and lack of conclusive evidence for its efficacy.

Patients who do not respond to conventional treatment sometimes seek alternative therapies, such as herbal supplements, ozone therapy, and hyperbaric oxygen therapy. These treatments are often promoted by practitioners outside mainstream medicine.

The efficacy and safety of alternative treatments are largely unproven and can pose risks. Patients pursuing these options may also face financial burdens due to the often high cost and lack of insurance coverage.

Guidelines and Recommendations:

Different medical organizations provide varying guidelines on Lyme disease treatment. The IDSA advocates for evidence-based, short-term antibiotic therapy, while the International Lyme and Associated Diseases Society (ILADS) supports individualized treatment plans, which may include longer courses of antibiotics.

These conflicting guidelines create confusion among healthcare providers and patients, complicating decision-making and care continuity.

Ethical and Legal Considerations in Lyme Disease Care.

The controversies in Lyme disease diagnosis and treatment raise important ethical and legal questions.

Ethical care requires that patients are fully informed about the benefits and risks of different treatment options. This is particularly challenging in the context of Lyme disease, where debates and conflicting guidelines can make it difficult for patients to understand their choices.

Ensuring that patients can make autonomous decisions about their care, while providing clear and balanced information, is a critical ethical responsibility for healthcare providers.

Disputes over treatment approaches can impact insurance coverage. Prolonged antibiotic treatments and alternative therapies are often not covered by insurance, limiting access for patients who believe these treatments are necessary for their recovery.

Legal battles have ensued over insurance denials and the right to pursue specific treatments, highlighting the need for policies that balance evidence-based practice with patient needs.

Regulatory and Legal Issues:

The regulation of diagnostic tests and treatments for Lyme disease is another contentious area. Stricter regulation aims to ensure safety and efficacy, but overly stringent policies may limit access to innovative diagnostic methods and experimental treatments.

Legal cases involving malpractice claims and disputes over treatment standards reflect the ongoing tensions within the medical community and underscore the complexity of providing care for Lyme disease patients.

The controversies and debates surrounding Lyme disease are deeply rooted in scientific, medical, and ethical complexities. The chronic Lyme disease controversy, disputes over treatment approaches, and ethical and legal considerations highlight the challenges faced by patients, healthcare providers, and policymakers.

Addressing these issues requires continued research, open dialogue, and a balanced approach to care that prioritizes patient well-being while adhering to rigorous scientific standards.

Through collaborative efforts and informed policy decisions, the goal is to improve the understanding, diagnosis, and treatment of Lyme disease, ultimately enhancing outcomes for all affected individuals.

www.ingramcontent.com/pod-product-compliance
Lightning Source LLC
Chambersburg PA
CBHW050235230526
45470CB00005B/1971